I0703348

ASHLEY WOODS

Homemade Natural Skincare

Crafting Simple and Effective Skincare Solutions at Home

Copyright © 2024 by Ashley Woods

All rights reserved. No part of this publication may be reproduced, stored or transmitted in any form or by any means, electronic, mechanical, photocopying, recording, scanning, or otherwise without written permission from the publisher. It is illegal to copy this book, post it to a website, or distribute it by any other means without permission.

First edition

This book was professionally typeset on Reedsy.
Find out more at reedsy.com

Contents

Introduction   1

Safety Information   3

Our Skin   5

Basic Ingredients   7

Basic Equipment   10

Basic Recipes   12

Cleaners   13

    Balancing Cleanser   13

    Honey and Green Tea Cleanser   14

    Rosehip and Chamomile Cleansing Balm   15

Scrubs   17

    Honey Oat Facial Scrub   17

    Versatile Body Scrub   18

    Coffee Body Scrub   19

Toners and Mists   20

    Green Tea and Witch Hazel Toner   20

    Apple Cider Vinegar and Aloe Toner   21

    Cucumber Mint Facial Mist   22

Masks   24

    Avocado and Honey Mask   24

    Oatmeal and Yogurt Mask   25

    Pumpkin and Honey Mask   26

Balms and Salves   27

    Basic Lip Balm   27

    Hand and Foot Balm   28

Skin Healing Salve   29

Chest Rub   31

Creams and Lotion Bars   33

Oil-free Cream   33

After Sun Cream   34

Solid Lotion or Massage Bars   36

Conclusion   38

Appendix   40

References   42

Introduction

If you are like me, you may have spent thousands of dollars over the years trying hundreds of products that all boast results that seem too good to be true. We are inundated with ads showing us heavily made up and retouched models meant to appear natural and flawless. When we examine the lists of ingredients on these products, we find things we cannot pronounce, let alone know where they come from or what purpose they have in our skincare. It's as if the goal is to make us believe that effective products must be meticulously formulated in a lab and carry that research and development price tag directly to you, the consumer.

But what if I told you that with some simple household ingredients – some you may already have in your pantry – you too can develop your own effective skincare solutions for pennies on the dollar? Imagine the sense of accomplishment and empowerment you'll feel when you see the results of your own creations on your skin.

In these pages, we will explore the basics and the benefits of simplifying your skincare routine. We are going to use natural plant-powered ingredients that you can pronounce. We will formulate luxurious products that can turn any average day into a spa day at home for a fraction of the cost. Most importantly, we will build your confidence because you *can* do this. Whether you have a PhD in DIY or you are a curious beginner, there is something in these chapters that you can learn and build on.

In addition to the easy-to-follow recipes in this book, we will also cover the basics of our body's largest organ–our skin, the properties and benefits of various ingredients, the fundamentals of formulation, and testing and adjusting your own recipes safely.

Now, if you are ready to dive in, let's get started!

Safety Information

The recipes and information provided in this book are intended for educational purposes only. While every effort has been made to ensure the accuracy and safety of the formulations, it is important to understand that skincare ingredients can vary in potency and individual skin reactions may occur.

Before using any homemade skincare product, it is strongly recommended that you perform a patch test on a small area of skin to check for allergic reactions or sensitivities. Stop using the product immediately if irritation occurs, and consult with a healthcare professional if necessary.

Furthermore, it is imperative to follow proper hygiene practices when preparing and storing homemade skincare products to prevent contamination and bacterial growth. Ensure that all equipment and containers are clean and sanitized before use.

The author and publisher of this book cannot be held liable for any adverse reactions, injuries, or damages resulting from the use of homemade skincare products. Users assume full responsibility for their skincare formulations and are encouraged to conduct thorough research and seek professional advice when needed.

By using the recipes and information provided in this book, you acknowledge and accept the inherent risks associated with DIY skincare and agree to use these formulations at your discretion.

Our Skin

When it comes to our skin, there is much more than meets the eye. Our skin is our body's largest organ, and it is extremely complex and hardworking. It is our first line of defense from pathogens and environmental factors we come into contact with in the outside world, and it is packed with nerves, blood vessels, hair follicles, proteins, fats, and minerals.

We have three layers to our skin:

1. Epidermis, the outer layer
2. Dermis, the middle layer
3. Hypodermis, the innermost layer

For our purposes of formulating our own skincare, the epidermis is what we are primarily concerned with. Our outermost layer of skin is constantly turning over dead skin cells with new ones, and it needs help to do this. When the skin's water content is low, our bodies have a difficult time with cell turnover. This means that hydrating the skin is crucial to skin health, both by drinking enough water and with moisturizing ingredients.

Moisturizing ingredients can also be divided into categories:

Moisturizing ingredients can also be divided into categories:

• Humectants

Humectants attract water.
Common natural humectant ingredients include honey, hyaluronic acid, and glycerin (glycerol).

• Occlusives

Heavier ingredients that prevent moisture loss.
Common, natural occlusives include beeswax, shea butter, and cocoa butter.

• Emollients

Lighter texture than occlusives and work as a barrier to protect the skin.
Common examples include cold-pressed oils like jojoba, almond, and argan oils.

While restoring moisture and preventing moisture loss are paramount to skin health, there are other products we can use to aid our skin's natural processes. Periodically, manual exfoliation with scrubs can help remove dead skin cells and improve the efficacy of our moisturizers and other products.

Basic Ingredients

You may be surprised that stocking your skincare 'pantry' may look a lot like stocking your kitchen pantry. In fact, this book contains several recipes that you can whip up without spending a dime.

My focus is on simple, effective, affordable, and *accessible* skincare for everyone. You certainly do not need all of these ingredients on hand, but having 2 to 3 in each category will make for a well-stocked skincare pantry.

I would like you to start thinking about your skin as an extension of your internal system. If it is something you would not put *in* your body, think twice before putting *on* your body.

Organic, minimally processed, sustainably grown, and ethically harvested ingredients are great if they are available to you. If not, choose the highest quality ingredients in your budget. You are worth it!

Oils:

- Jojoba oil
- Sweet almond oil
- Argan oil

- Rosehip oil
- Coconut oil
- Olive oil
- Avocado oil

Butters:

- Shea butter
- Cocoa butter
- Mango butter

Exfoliants:

- Sugars
- Salts
- Ground coffee
- Ground grains (oats, rice, etc.)

Other additives:

- Beeswax
- Honey
- Plain yogurt
- Apple cider vinegar
- Aloe vera gel
- Witch hazel
- Rose water
- Brewed herbal teas and infusions

Essential oils:

- Lavender
- Rosemary
- Tea tree
- Peppermint

The list of essential oils is virtually endless. You can find many resources online about their properties and benefits. The most important thing I want to remind you of is that essential oils are highly concentrated and should always be properly diluted before being applied to your skin.

If you are pregnant, nursing, or have medical conditions, consult a healthcare professional before using essential oils topically. Some oils are unsafe for certain conditions or may interact with certain medications.

Before using any homemade skincare product, it is strongly recommended that you perform a patch test on a small area of skin to check for allergic reactions or sensitivities. Stop using the product immediately if irritation occurs, and consult with a healthcare professional if necessary.

Basic Equipment

If you have ever baked a cake or made a meal at home, you will likely have most of the equipment you'll need to craft your own skincare in your kitchen. I always opt for non-reactive tools and equipment, which means that they are made from materials that will not react with acidic or alkaline ingredients. Stainless steel, glass, and ceramics are all non-reactive materials. Avoid using plastics that can absorb some of our more intense ingredients, such as essential oils.

You will need:

- Mixing bowls
- Measuring cups and spoons
- Whisks
- Mixing spoons/scrapers
- Wire mesh strainer
- Double boiler — Making a double boiler for melting solid butters and waxes with a heat-proof bowl over a pan of simmering water is easy.
- Containers for your finished products — Dark glass jars or bottles will extend the life of your products but are not required. Mason jars, tins, or repurposing empty containers that you have cleaned and sanitized work as well.

- Labels — Use waterproof labels and include the date you made your product.
- Digital scale — A helpful tool for precise measurements.
- Funnel — It can make packaging your liquid ingredients easier.
- Notebook — Making notes as you craft your own products will help you refine and develop your recipes in the future. Noting things like substitutions and what you liked or didn't like about your finished product will be invaluable information.

Basic Recipes

As we get into recipes, I want to keep the ingredients and techniques simple. We do not need to overcomplicate our skincare routines, and I want to empower you to make substitutions as you see fit and test these recipes for yourself.

When it comes to substitutions, the simplest things to consider are the forms of ingredients. For example, you would not want to substitute a liquid oil for a solid plant butter if you were making a balm, as it would not be solid at room temperature. Other things to consider when substituting are your skin type, allergies, sensitivities, and fragrances.

It's worth noting that these recipes are designed to make small batches of product. This is because, in natural skincare, many of the ingredients we use can spoil over time. By making small batches, we ensure our products are as fresh as possible, as these recipes don't contain preservatives or stabilizing ingredients. This underscores the importance of sterilizing our equipment and maintaining proper hygiene.

Now, let's get to the good part!

Cleaners

Balancing Cleanser

This is an excellent cleanser for oily or acne-prone skin

- ¼ cup liquid castile soap (unscented)
- 2 Tbsp pure aloe vera gel
- 1 Tbsp argan oil
- 10 drops tea tree essential oil

Mix all ingredients in a small bowl, stirring until well combined.

Transfer to an airtight container for storage.

To use, wet your skin with lukewarm water. Use a small amount of cleanser and massage it into your skin. Allow the cleanser to sit for 1-2 minutes before rinsing thoroughly. Avoid your eyes.

Benefits:

- Tea tree oil is naturally antibacterial and anti-inflammatory.
- Aloe vera gel is soothing and hydrating.

- Argan oil is non-comedogenic, meaning it will not clog pores, and provides moisture without feeling greasy.
- Castile soap is a gentle cleanser made from vegetable oils.

Honey and Green Tea Cleanser

This cleanser has benefits for combination skin

- 1 Tbsp raw honey
- 1 Tbsp brewed green tea (let cool to room temperature)
- 1 tsp jojoba oil
- 1 tsp unscented liquid castile soap (optional)

Brew green tea and allow it to cool.

Mix all ingredients in a small bowl, stirring until well combined.

If you prefer suds or need more cleansing action, add the liquid castile soap and stir until incorporated.

Transfer to an airtight container for storage.

To use, wet your skin with lukewarm water. Use a small amount of cleaner and massage it into your skin. Allow the cleanser to sit for 1-2 minutes before rinsing thoroughly. Avoid your eyes.

Benefits:

- Honey is naturally antibacterial and a humectant which draws

moisture into the skin.
- Green tea contains antioxidants and is anti-inflammatory.
- Jojoba oil is similar to the sebum our skin produces and can help balance combination skin.
- Castile soap is a gentle cleanser made from vegetable oils.

Rosehip and Chamomile Cleansing Balm

This cleanser works well on mature or dry skin. It is also effective as a makeup remover and travel-friendly as a solid.

- 1 Tbsp rosehip seed oil
- 1 Tbsp shea butter
- 1 Tbsp beeswax pellets
- 1 Tbsp dried chamomile flowers

In a double boiler or a heat-safe bowl, combine all ingredients.

Place the double boiler, or bowl, over a pot of simmering water and gently heat until the shea butter and beeswax pellets are melted, stirring occasionally until well combined.

Remove from heat and strain.

Transfer to an airtight container for storage.

To use, apply a small amount of cleaner to your face and massage it into your skin, focusing on areas with makeup. Wet your hands and continue massaging the balm into your skin. Rinse thoroughly.

Benefits:

- Rosehip seed oil is anti-inflammatory and rich in vitamins A, C, and E.
- Shea butter is non-comedogenic and very moisturizing.
- Beeswax is a natural emulsifier that allows solid and liquid ingredients to blend smoothly. It can also provide a protective barrier on the skin and lock in moisture.
- Chamomile is soothing for sensitive or irritated skin and is anti-inflammatory.

Scrubs

Honey Oat Facial Scrub

A simple scrub gentle enough for your face

- 2 Tbsp rolled oats
- 1 Tbsp honey
- 1 Tbsp plain yogurt (optional)

Grind your oats into a coarse powder using a blender, food processor, or mortar and pestle.

Mix all ingredients in a small bowl, stirring until well combined.

You can adjust the consistency by adding a little water if the mixture is too thick or adding more ground oats if the mixture is too thin.

Transfer to an airtight container for storage.

To use, wet your skin with lukewarm water. Use a small amount of scrub and massage it into your skin for 1-2 minutes before rinsing thoroughly. Avoid your eyes.

Benefits:

- Oats are soothing on irritated skin and a gentle manual exfoliator.
- Honey is naturally antibacterial and a humectant which draws moisture into the skin.
- Yogurt will add additional moisture and contains lactic acid, which helps gently exfoliate the skin.

Versatile Body Scrub

This body scrub is highly customizable and takes minutes to prepare

- 1 cup granulated sugar (white or brown)
- ½ cup carrier oil (coconut oil, olive oil, almond oil, etc.)
- 10-15 drops essential oils (optional)

Mix all ingredients in a small bowl, stirring until well combined.

Transfer to an airtight container for storage.

To use, wet your skin with water. Apply scrub to one area of your body at a time and massage into your skin using circular motions. Focus on joints and other rough or dry areas. Avoid any sensitive areas, wounds, or broken skin.

Use caution if using in the bath or shower as the oils can make the floor of your bath or shower slippery.

Coffee Body Scrub

This scrub's scent is invigorating for coffee lovers and can help temporarily boost circulation

- ½ cup ground coffee
- ½ cup granulated sugar (white or brown)
- ¼ cup carrier oil (coconut oil, olive oil, almond oil, etc.)

Mix all ingredients in a small bowl, stirring until well combined.

Transfer to an airtight container for storage.

To use, wet your skin with water. Apply scrub to one area of your body at a time and massage into your skin using circular motions. Focus on joints and other rough or dry areas. Avoid any sensitive areas, wounds, or broken skin.

Use caution if using in the bath or shower, as the oil can make the floor of your bath or shower slippery.

Benefits:

- Coffee, when ground, is a great natural exfoliant and does not dissolve like salt and sugar scrubs. The caffeine in coffee can help temporarily improve circulation and tighten the skin.

Toners and Mists

Green Tea and Witch Hazel Toner

This is a toner for all skin types

- 1 cup brewed green tea
- 2 Tbsp witch hazel
- 5 drops tea tree oil (optional)

Brew green tea and allow it to cool.

Combine ingredients in a clean bottle. Shake well to mix.

To use, apply the toner to your face using a cotton ball or pad. Let the toner dry before following with your moisturizer.

This toner can also be used as a refreshing facial mist if your bottle has an atomizer and you store it in the fridge.

Benefits:

- Green tea contains antioxidants and is anti-inflammatory.

- Witch hazel is astringent, which helps tighten the skin and reduce pore size.
- Tea tree oil is naturally antibacterial and anti-inflammatory.

Apple Cider Vinegar and Aloe Toner

This toner helps balance the pH of the skin

- ⅓ cup apple cider vinegar
- ⅔ cup distilled water
- 2 Tbsp pure aloe vera gel
- 3-5 drops lavender essential oil (optional)

Combine ingredients in a clean bottle. Shake well to mix.

To use, apply the toner to your face using a cotton ball or pad. Let the toner dry before following with your moisturizer.

This toner can also be used as a refreshing facial mist if your bottle has an atomizer and you store it in the fridge.

Note: Using distilled water is essential in your skincare formulations because tap, filtered, or boiled water may still contain undesirable microorganisms or trace minerals.

Benefits:

- Apple cider vinegar is acidic and helps balance the skin's pH. The malic acid in apple cider vinegar can also help lighten dark spots over time and even skin tone.

- Aloe vera gel is soothing and hydrating.
- Lavender essential oil in this formulation, or other essential oils of your choice, can help mask the vinegar's fragrance if it is too intense.

Cucumber Mint Facial Mist

This facial mist is cooling and refreshing

- ½ fresh cucumber
- 1 handful of fresh mint leaves
- 1 cup distilled water
- 1 Tbsp witch hazel

Peel and chop the cucumber into small pieces.

Add the cucumber, mint leaves, and distilled water to a blender, blending until smooth.

Add the witch hazel to the mixture and stir until combined.

Strain the mixture into a clean bottle with an atomizer and store in the refrigerator.

To use, remove the bottle from the fridge and shake well. Mist your face and body as desired.

Note: Using distilled water is essential in your skincare formulations because tap, filtered, or boiled water may still contain undesirable microorganisms or trace minerals.

Benefits:

- Cucumbers have a high water content, making them moisturizing. They also have natural cooling properties and can soothe irritated skin.
- Mint possesses natural antibacterial properties, is cooling, and can help control excess oil production in the skin.
- Witch hazel is astringent, which helps tighten the skin and reduce pore size.

Masks

Avocado and Honey Mask

This is a deeply hydrating and soothing mask

- ½ ripe avocado
- 1 Tbsp raw honey

Mash the avocado in a small bowl until smooth.

Add honey and stir to combine until it forms a smooth paste.

Store in the fridge in an airtight container and use within 1-2 days.

To use, apply the mask to clean dry skin using your fingers or brush, avoiding the eye area. Leave on for 10-20 minutes. Rinse your skin with lukewarm water.

Benefits:

- Avocado is rich in nourishing oils as well as vitamins A, D, and E.
- Honey is naturally antibacterial and a humectant which draws

moisture into the skin.

Oatmeal and Yogurt Mask

This mask is very soothing to irritated or sensitive skin

- 2 Tbsp plain yogurt
- 1 Tbsp rolled oats
- 1 tsp raw honey

Grind your oats into a fine powder using a blender, food processor, or mortar and pestle.

Mix all ingredients in a small bowl, creating a smooth paste.

Store in the fridge in an airtight container and use within 1-2 days.

To use, apply the mask to clean dry skin using your fingers or brush, avoiding the eye area. Leave on for 10-20 minutes. Rinse your skin with lukewarm water.

Benefits:

- Yogurt will add additional moisture and contains lactic acid, which helps gently exfoliate the skin.
- Oats are anti-inflammatory and calm redness or irritation of the skin
- Honey is naturally antibacterial and a humectant which draws moisture into the skin.

Pumpkin and Honey Mask

This mask helps brighten and moisturize the skin

- ¼ cup pumpkin puree
- 1 Tbsp raw honey
- 1 Tbsp plain yogurt

Mix all ingredients in a small bowl, creating a smooth paste.

Store in the fridge in an airtight container and use within 1-2 days.

To use, apply the mask to clean dry skin using your fingers or brush, avoiding the eye area. Leave on for 10-20 minutes. Rinse your skin with lukewarm water.

Benefits:

- Pumpkin is rich in enzymes, alpha-hydroxy-acids (AHAs), and vitamins that brighten and rejuvenate the skin.
- Honey is naturally antibacterial and a humectant which draws moisture into the skin.
- Yogurt will add additional moisture and contains lactic acid, which helps gently exfoliate.

Balms and Salves

Basic Lip Balm

An all-purpose lip balm to restore and maintain moisture

- 1 Tbsp beeswax pellets
- 2 Tbsp coconut oil
- 1 Tbsp shea butter
- 1-2 drops peppermint or rosemary essential oil (optional)

In a double boiler or a heat-safe bowl, combine all ingredients except the essential oils.

Place the double boiler, or bowl, over a pot of simmering water and gently heat until the beeswax pellets, coconut oil, and shea butter are melted, stirring occasionally until well combined.

Remove from heat and add essential oils, if using. Stir well to combine.

Carefully pour the mixture into lip balm tubes, small jars, or tins for storage.

Allow your balm to cool completely and solidify before sealing your containers.

To use, apply to your lips as needed to maintain moisture and prevent dryness or cracking.

Benefits:

- Beeswax provides a protective barrier to prevent moisture loss.
- Coconut oil is rich in fatty acids and has moisturizing and softening properties.
- Shea butter is deeply moisturizing and contains vitamins A and E, which promote skin healing.

Hand and Foot Balm

A versatile balm for rough hands and feet

- ¼ cup beeswax pellets
- ¼ cup shea butter
- 2 oz avocado oil
- 10 drops essential oils such as lavender and/or peppermint

In a double boiler or a heat-safe bowl, combine all ingredients except the essential oils.

Place the double boiler, or bowl, over a pot of simmering water and gently heat until the beeswax pellets and shea butter are melted, stirring occasionally until well combined.

Remove from heat and add ten drops of essential oil(s) if using. Stir well to combine.

Carefully pour the mixture into small jars or tins for storage.

Allow your balm to cool completely and solidify before sealing your containers.

To use, apply a small amount to your hands, feet, or other rough areas as needed, massaging into the skin until absorbed.

Benefits:

- Beeswax provides a protective barrier to prevent moisture loss.
- Shea butter is deeply moisturizing and contains vitamins A and E, which promote skin healing.
- Avocado oil is rich in vitamins A, D, and E and helps nourish and hydrate the skin.

Skin Healing Salve

A multipurpose salve for minor cuts, scrapes, or insect bites

- ½ cup chamomile infused oil
- 2 Tbsp cocoa butter
- 2 Tbsp coconut oil
- 2 Tbsp beeswax pellets
- 10 drops tea tree oil

Prepare your chamomile-infused oil by combining 2 Tbsp dried chamomile flowers with ½ cup of your preferred carrier oil (jojoba, almond oil, olive oil, etc.) in a saucepan or double boiler.

Gently heat your oil on very low heat for one hour to infuse.

Strain the solids from your oil infusion with a wire mesh strainer.

In a double boiler or a heat-safe bowl, combine all ingredients except the tea tree oil.

Place the double boiler, or bowl, over a pot of simmering water and gently heat until the chamomile infused oil, cocoa butter, coconut oil, and beeswax pellets are melted, stirring occasionally until well combined.

Remove from heat and add tea tree oil. Stir well to combine.

Carefully pour the mixture into small jars or tins for storage.

Allow your salve to cool completely and solidify before sealing your containers.

To use, apply a small amount to problem areas, such as minor cuts, scrapes, or insect bites, and reapply as needed.

Benefits:

- Chamomile soothes irritated skin and is anti-inflammatory.
- Cocoa butter is moisturizing and has antioxidants that help repair the skin.

- Coconut oil has antimicrobial and anti-inflammatory properties.
- Beeswax provides a protective barrier to prevent moisture loss and helps solidify your salve.
- Tea tree oil has antimicrobial, antifungal, and anti-inflammatory properties.

Chest Rub

A classic recipe to help relieve chest and upper respiratory congestion

- ½ cup coconut oil
- 2 Tbsp beeswax pellets
- 10 drops eucalyptus essential oil
- 10 drops peppermint essential oil
- 10 drops rosemary essential oil

In a double boiler or a heat-safe bowl, combine all ingredients except the essential oils.

Place the double boiler, or bowl, over a pot of simmering water and gently heat until the coconut oil and beeswax pellets are melted, stirring occasionally until well combined.

Remove from heat and add essential oils, stirring well to combine.

Carefully pour the mixture into small jars or tins for storage.

Allow your balm to cool completely and solidify before sealing your containers.

To use, apply a small amount to your chest, massaging in circular motions. Avoid applying too close to your nose, mouth, and eyes.

Benefits:

- Coconut oil is a moisturizer and acts as a solid base for this rub.
- Beeswax provides a protective barrier to prevent moisture loss from the skin and helps solidify this formulation.
- Eucalyptus oil has decongestant properties to help ease breathing.
- Peppermint oil contains menthol and has cooling properties.
- Rosemary oil has anti-inflammatory and decongestant properties.

Creams and Lotion Bars

Oil-free Cream

This lightweight cream uses water-based ingredients

- ½ cup shea butter
- ¼ cup pure aloe vera gel
- 2 Tbsp vegetable glycerin
- 1 Tbsp cornstarch
- 5-10 drops essential oils for fragrance (optional)

In a double boiler or a heat-safe bowl, add the shea butter.

Place the double boiler, or bowl, over a pot of simmering water and gently heat until the shea butter is melted.

Remove from heat and add the aloe vera, vegetable glycerin, and cornstarch, stirring well to combine. Make sure there are no lumps, and the mixture is smooth.

Add 5-10 drops of your favorite essential oils, if using, stirring well to combine.

Allow the mixture to cool for 10 minutes or until it begins to solidify around the edges of your bowl.

Using a stand mixer, hand mixer, or whisk, whip the mixture for 5-10 minutes until it becomes light and fluffy.

Transfer to an airtight container for storage. Ensure that your cream is cooled entirely before sealing your containers.

To use, apply to your skin as needed, massaging until absorbed.

Benefits:

- Shea butter is deeply moisturizing and non-comedogenic, which will not clog your pores.
- Aloe vera is soothing, hydrating, and lightweight.
- Glycerin is non-comedogenic and a humectant which draws moisture into the skin.
- Cornstarch acts as a thickener and improves the texture of the cream.

After Sun Cream

This rich, soothing cream is perfect for sunburns

- ½ cup shea butter
- 2 Tbsp pure aloe vera gel
- 2 Tbsp kukui nut oil or argan oil
- 5 drops lavender oil

- 5 drops peppermint oil

In a double boiler or a heat-safe bowl, add the shea butter and kukui nut oil.

Place the double boiler, or bowl, over a pot of simmering water and gently heat until the shea butter is melted.

Remove from heat and add the aloe vera and essential oils, stirring well to combine.

Allow the mixture to cool for 10 minutes or until it begins to solidify around the edges of your bowl.

Using a stand mixer, hand mixer, or whisk, whip the mixture for 5-10 minutes until it becomes light and fluffy.

Transfer to an airtight container for storage. Ensure that your cream is cooled entirely before sealing your containers.

To use, apply liberally to your skin as needed, massaging until absorbed.

Benefits:

- Shea butter is deeply moisturizing and contains vitamins A and E, which promote skin healing.
- Aloe vera is soothing and hydrating.
- Kukui nut oil has anti-inflammatory properties and contains vitamins A, C, and E.
- Lavender oil is calming and can relieve itching.
- Peppermint oil contains menthol and has cooling properties.

Solid Lotion or Massage Bars

This highly customizable recipe creates solid moisturizing bars ideal for travel

- ½ cup cocoa butter
- ¼ cup carrier oil (jojoba oil, olive oil, almond oil, etc.)
- ¼ cup beeswax pellets
- 10 drops essential oils (optional for fragrance)

In a double boiler or a heat-safe bowl, combine all ingredients except the essential oils.

Place the double boiler, or bowl, over a pot of simmering water and gently heat until the cocoa butter, oil, and beeswax pellets are melted, stirring occasionally until well combined.

Remove from heat and add essential oils, if using, stirring well to combine.

Carefully pour the mixture into silicone molds or another form for your desired shape.

Allow the bars to cool completely before releasing them from the mold.

Store in a tin or airtight container.

To use, rub the solid bar between your hands or on your skin, allowing your body heat to melt it. Apply as much or as little as you like, massaging until absorbed.

Benefits:

- Cocoa butter is deeply moisturizing and solid at room temperature.
- Beeswax provides a protective barrier to prevent moisture loss and helps solidify your bars.
- Carrier oils have different benefits, and some absorb into the skin faster. Choose a lighter oil, like jojoba or almond oil, for a less greasy feel. Choose a heavier oil, like olive or avocado oil, that absorbs less quickly for massage bars.

Conclusion

When it comes to skincare, the journey towards healthier, more radiant skin begins with the empowering decision to take control of your skincare routine. As we conclude this exploration into crafting your own skincare, it becomes evident that the power to nurture and rejuvenate our skin lies quite literally in our hands.

Throughout this book, we have explored an array of natural ingredients, from soothing aloe vera to nourishing avocado oil, discovering only some of their remarkable properties and benefits they can have on our skin. By harnessing the power of ingredients in our own kitchens, we have discovered skincare formulations that are not only effective but also gentle and sustainable.

Beyond the tangible benefits of do-it-yourself skincare, there is a profound connection to oneself and to the natural world that emerges. Crafting our own skincare offers a sense of empowerment, empowering us to become active participants in our own wellness journey. It fosters a sense of creativity and experimentation, encouraging us to explore new ingredients, adapt recipes to suit our unique needs, and tailor skincare rituals that resonate with our personal preferences.

Let's not just absorb the knowledge and inspiration from these pages, but put it into action. Embrace the beauty of simplicity, prioritize quality over quantity, and cultivate a mindful approach to skincare that respects both our bodies and the planet. We've only scratched the surface of the possibilities with a short list of basic ingredients. This is just the beginning of your journey into formulating your own skincare.

Happy crafting!

Appendix

Common Skincare Oils	Comedogenic Rating
Argan Oil	0
Hemp Seed Oil	0
Castor Oil	1
Grapeseed Oil	1
Rosehip Oil	1
Jojoba Oil	2
Kukui Nut Oil	2
Olive Oil	2
Sweet Almond Oil	2
Evening Primrose Oil	2-3
Avocado Oil	3
Coconut Oil	4

Common Skincare Butters	Comedogenic Rating
Shea Butter	0-2
Mango Butter	2
Kokum Butter	2
Cocoa Butter	4

Essential Oil Dilution %	Essential Oil Amount	Carrier Oil Amount
0.5%	1 drop	2 teaspoons
1%	1 drop	1 teaspoon
2%	2 drops	1 teaspoon
3%	3 drops	1 teaspoon
5%	5 drops	1 teaspoon

References

The Healthline Editorial Team. (2018, December 19). *Epidermis function: Get to know your skin.* Healthline. https://www.healthline.com/health/epidermis-function

AromaWeb. (n.d.). *Essential Oils Directory: Essential Oil Properties, Uses and Benefits.* Retrieved May 30, 2024, from https://www.aromaweb.com/essentialoils/index.php

Hernandez, P. (2023, December 6). *Oils and Butters Comedogenic Rating List | Oh mighty health.* Oh Mighty Health. https://ohmightyhealth.com/comedogenic-rating-list/

Professional, C. C. M. (n.d.). *Skin.* Cleveland Clinic. https://my.clevelandclinic.org/health/body/10978-skin

Wade, G. (2019, December 6). *Skincare 101: The science behind your favorite moisturizers, serums, actives, and more.* Popular Science. https://www.popsci.com/story/health/best-skincare-routine-ingredient-chemistry-science/

www.ingramcontent.com/pod-product-compliance
Lightning Source LLC
Chambersburg PA
CBHW061314250726
48653CB00002B/932